Gout

(Severe Form of Arthritis)

Dr. Sheila Harrison

Disclaimer

This content serves to provide general information about the disease and aims to empower you to seek prompt medical assistance if necessary to prevent complications. It's essential to stress that this information is not a substitute for consulting a qualified physician. The field of medical science is continually evolving, and due to the dynamic nature of medical knowledge, we recommend seeking expert advice if you encounter any inconsistencies or intend to take action based on the information in this content. Never disregard professional medical guidance or delay treatment based on something you've read online, including this material, or from any other online source. Always remember that the internet cannot cure you; rather, healing comes through the guidance of medical professionals and the providence of God.

Table of Contents

Overview (Gout)

Gout is a painful form of arthritis. Arthritis is a disease which causes pain and swelling in the joints, and the most common types of arthritis include osteoarthritis and rheumatoid arthritis.

When your body has extra uric acid, sharp crystals can form in your joints (usually your big toe). Flare-ups of symptoms like pain and swelling come and go in periods called gout attacks. Treatment is usually a combination of symptom management and changing your diet

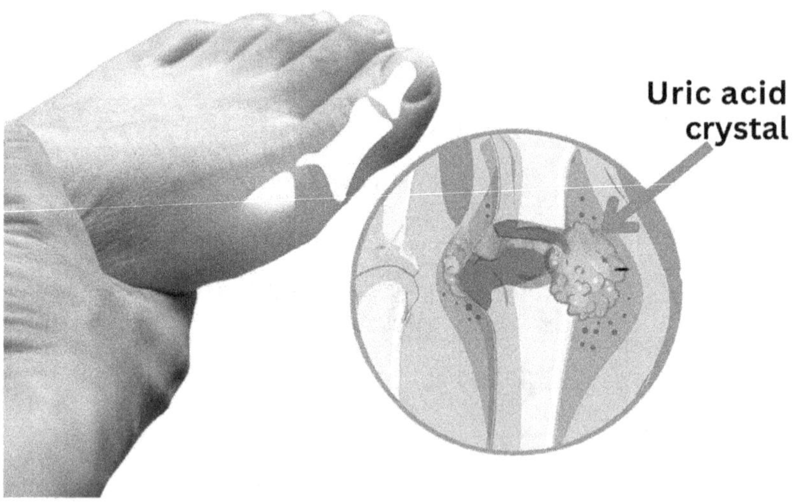

Section 1
What is Gout?

Gout is a type of inflammatory arthritis that makes your joints hurt and swell. An increased uric acid buildup, or an excess of uric acid in the blood, can lead to gout. This condition is characterized by the accumulation of tiny crystals in the joints, which can cause discomfort, swelling, and difficulty moving the affected joints. These crystals of uric acid can also accumulate beneath our skin, forming elevated white nodules known as "gouty tophi."

A gout attack usually includes local swelling, heat, redness, and tenderness in a joint, especially in the foot, ankle, or knee. Some patients have fever and chills as the first warning that an attack of gout is coming on. The pain is caused by the crystals that form in and around the joints.

Gout is more common in men and the risk factor increases with age. It occurs in people who have high levels of urate (uric acid) in their blood. Despite this, having some uric acid in your bloodstream is no cause for concern. Our body creates urate daily as it breaks down purines. Purines are chemicals that are naturally created in our body but they are also present in some food that we eat. It is where uric acid originates from.

As urate increases, our body gets rid of all the excess through the kidneys and in our urine. The problem will only occur when our body is making too much uric acid or our kidneys are unable to get rid of enough of it. As the body fails to stabilize the level of urate, the crystals will begin to form. They mainly occur in and around firm joint tissues such as the cartilage. Crystals can also appear under the skin and may even occur in internal organs such as the kidneys.

Lifestyle choices are not the main reason why most people get gout. People always mistake overeating and drinking too much alcohol to be the main causes of gout. While this can make attacks of gout more likely, it is not always the case. On any day, about three-quarters of the uric acid in our system comes from the breakdown of purines produced within our body, while only about a quarter comes from the breakdown of purines in the food and drink we consume.

The big toe joint is the most usually affected by gout. However, it may impact more joints, such as your:

➢ Knees.

➢ Ankles.

➢ Feet.

➢ Hands

➢ Wrists.

➢ Elbows.

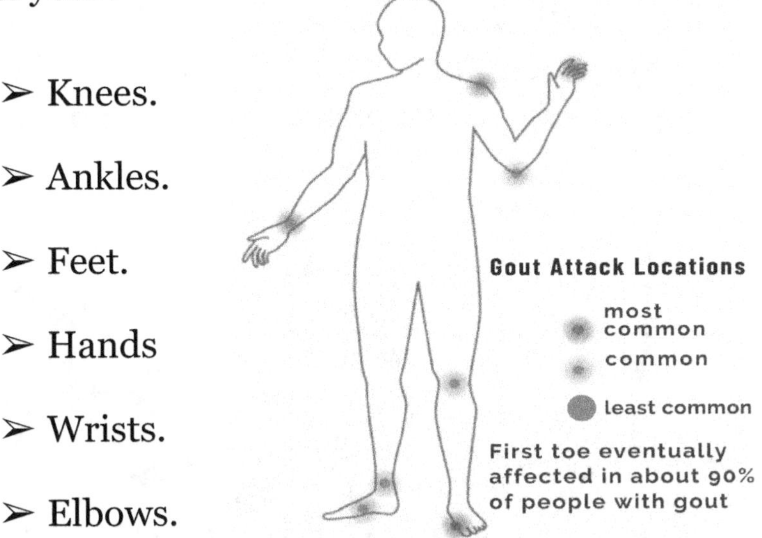

Gout symptoms come and go (recur) in episodes called flares or gout attacks. A healthcare provider will suggest medications and changes to your diet that will lower your uric acid levels and minimize how often you experience gout attacks in the future.

Globally, gout is becoming increasingly common, likely due to changes in diet around the world over recent years and an aging population.

The prevalence of gout is greater than 1% in most developed countries, including the USA (3.9%), Australia (5.2%), Canada (3.8%), Greece (4.75%), Germany (1.4%), and the UK (2.5%).

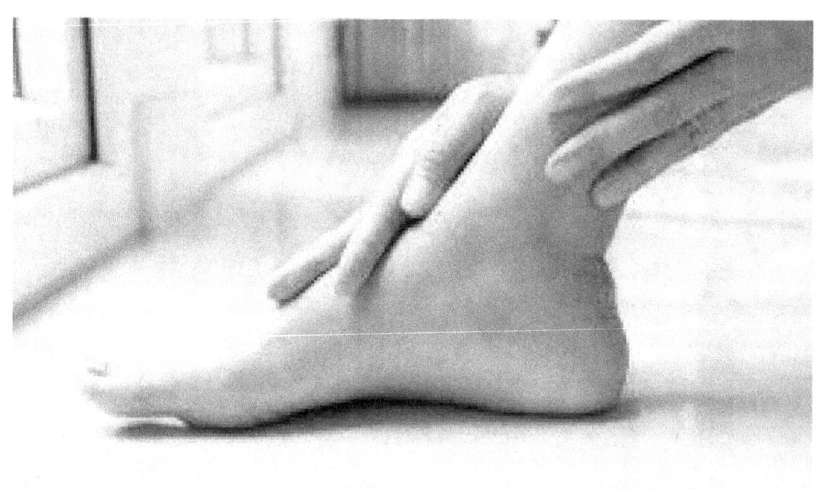

Section 2
Causes of Gout

A buildup of excess uric acid in your body(blood) causes gout.

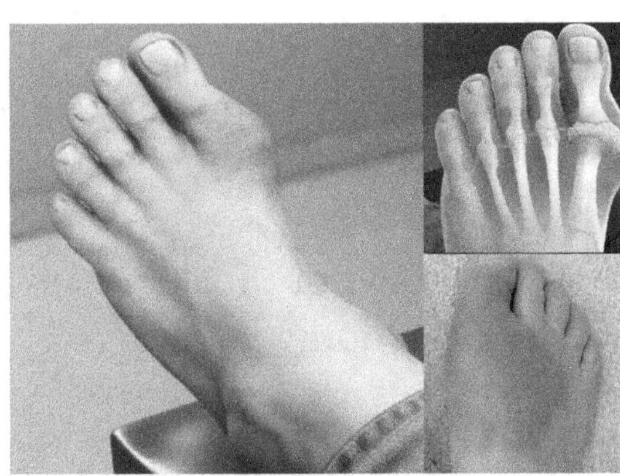

Your body naturally makes uric acid when it breaks down chemicals called purines found in certain foods and drinks. Your kidneys usually filter uric acid out of your blood, and then it leaves your body when you pee. Sometimes your body makes too much uric acid, or your kidneys don't remove it from your blood fast enough. When your body has high levels of uric acid (hyperuricemia), uric acid crystals can build up and settle into your joints. The sharp crystals clump together and cause sudden episodes of pain, swelling and other symptoms. Having temporarily high uric acid levels doesn't mean you'll definitely develop gout. Many people with hyperuricemia never get gout.

Risk Factors of Gout

Gout is caused by crystals building up in the joints, which is a normal and natural process brought on by an excess of uric acid in the blood.

Non-modifiable risk factors refer to those characteristics that increase an individual's risk of developing gout and cannot be altered. Modifiable risk factors are those that relate to our ability to control some of the elements that increase our risk of developing gout.

Modifiable Risk Factors

☑ Diet

When you are eating too many fatty meals like burgers and cola from fast-food chains, for instance, the body will struggle to eliminate uric acid naturally and gout can occur. Eating or drinking foods high in purines are more likely to lead to high uric acid levels in your body that cause gout, including:

> **Sugary drinks and sweets:** Standard table sugar is half fructose (fruit sugar), which breaks down into uric acid. Any food

or drink with high sugar content can trigger gout.

- ➤ **High fructose corn syrup:** This is a concentrated form of fructose. Packaged food products and processed snacks can contain lots of high fructose corn syrup.
- ➤ **Alcohol:** Even though not all alcoholic drinks are high in purines, alcohol prevents your kidneys from eliminating uric acid, pulling it back into your body, where it continues to accumulate. Having more than two alcoholic drinks per day also increases your risk.
- ➤ **Organ meats**: These include liver, tripe, sweetbreads, brains and kidneys.
- ➤ **Game meats:** Specialties such as goose, veal and venison all contain high levels of purines.
- ➤ **Certain seafood:** Herring, scallops, mussels, codfish, tuna, trout and haddock.
- ➤ **Red meat:** Beef, lamb, pork and bacon.
- ➤ **Turkey**: Especially processed deli turkey.
- ➤ Gravy and meat sauces.

☑ **Obesity**

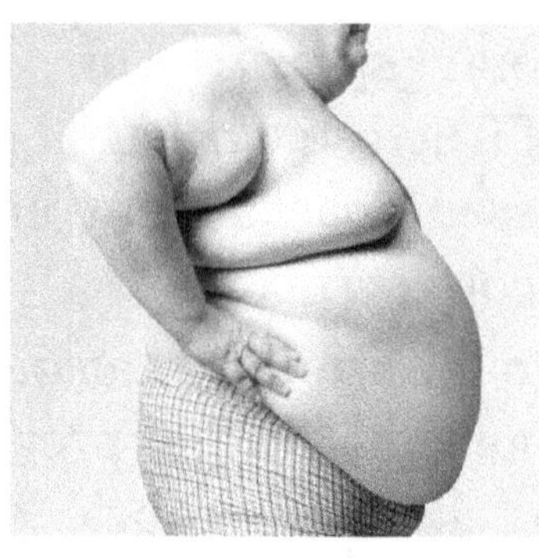

Being overweight increases your risk of gout, even with a relatively healthy diet. This is because your body produces more uric acid and your kidneys have a harder time processing and eliminating them. Excessive food intake increases the body's production of uric acid. The kidneys will have to work extra hard to eliminate it and increase the risk of a gout attack. A patient diagnosed with gout will be advised to make lifestyle changes that will enable him or her to lose weight.

Non-Modifiable Risk Factors

- ➤ **Family History:** Having a family member or Having a biological parent or grandparent who has gout puts us at a higher risk of developing gout.
- ➤ **Age:** Gout becomes more common as we get older, partially because we are more

likely to be affected by other illnesses as we age too.

➤ **Gender:** Often thought of as being a man's condition, gout affects over four times more men than women. Women may also develop the condition, but this usually only happens after menopause as estrogen released during the female reproductive cycle speeds up the removal of uric acid by the kidneys.

➤ **Racial Background:** People from African-Caribbean backgrounds are more likely to have gout than people of white European backgrounds, and the likelihood of having gout is much higher again in people from parts of South East Asia and Australasia.

➤ **Medication:** Diuretic medications taken to help lower high blood pressure can raise uric acid levels. Patients with rheumatoid arthritis or psoriasis who take drugs that suppress the immune system also have an increased risk of getting gout. If a patient is diagnosed with gout, a doctor might change their medications to ensure lower levels of uric acid. The use of other medications such as salicylates, cyclosporine, niacin and levodopa can also lead to gout.

The use of certain medications can cause a rise in uric acid levels. Some of these drugs may include;

- Low-dose aspirin
- Thiazide diuretics (commonly prescribed for hypertension)
- Diuretic medication (water pills),
- Immunosuppressants.

➤ **Medical Condition:** Gout tends to go hand-in-hand with other illnesses. Sometimes, having other illnesses makes it harder to treat gout or can mean that doctors have to be careful when choosing which medications to prescribe.

Recent hospital stay – Recent surgery or trauma has been associated with an increased risk of gout. This is because fluid levels often fluctuate during hospital stays, and patients might also be put on diuretics depending on the nature of their illnesses

People with certain health conditions are more likely to develop gout, including:

- Overweight or obesity.
- Congestive heart failure. (Cardiovascular diseases)
- Diabetes.
- Hypertension (high blood pressure).
- Kidney disease.
- Blood cancer.

When we are unwell or less able to be active, engaging a dedicated carer to visit us at home and assist with daily activities can be helpful.

Section 3
Symptoms of Gout

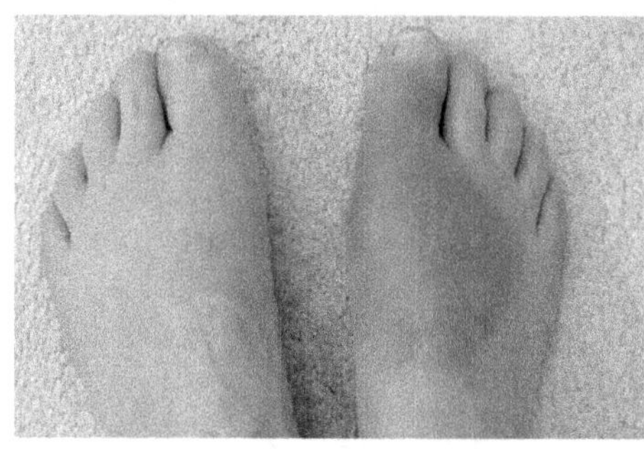

Gout usually causes red, swollen joints. The swelling might make the joints feel large, hot, and tight. Gout can be painful and affect people's lives and their ability to take care of themselves properly.

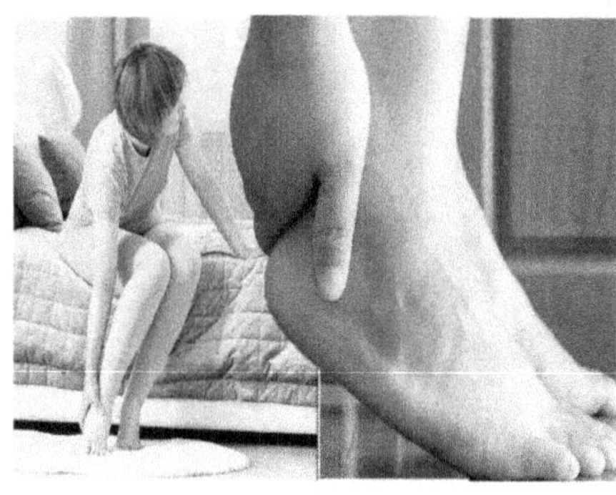

Joint pain is usually most severe within the first 4 to 12 hours, and the lingering discomfort may last from days to weeks afterwards. As gout progresses, you may not be able to move your joints normally.

The symptoms of gout can be similar to the symptoms of other conditions, which is why it's important to see a licensed healthcare professional for a definite diagnosis. Without an accurate diagnosis, you could get the wrong treatment which is likely to be ineffective or even harmful.

Section 4
Diagnosing Gout

Joint pain can arise from a number of conditions, so you should consult a licensed doctor for an assessment and to confirm a diagnosis.

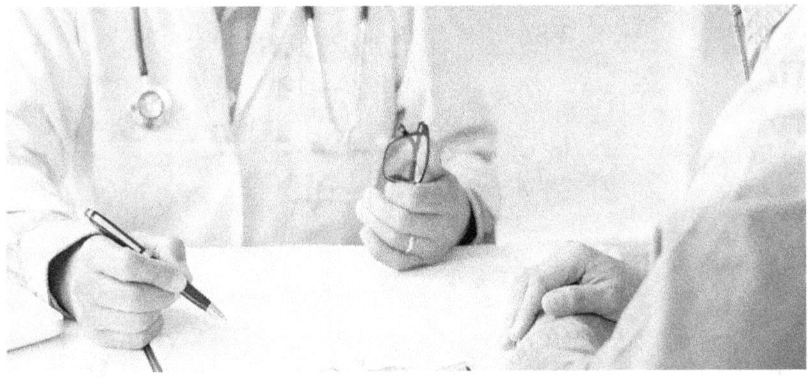

There are several different treatments available for gout so it's important to consult a medical professional, who can then create a tailored treatment plan for you.

To diagnose gout, a healthcare provider will diagnose gout with a physical exam. They'll ask you about your symptoms and examine your affected joints. Tell your provider when you first noticed symptoms like pain and swelling in your joint and how often the symptoms come and go.

Clinical Diagnostic testing options for gout

Your healthcare provider might use a few imaging tests to take pictures of your affected joints. These tests can also show if gout has caused any changes in your joints. You might need:

- X-rays.

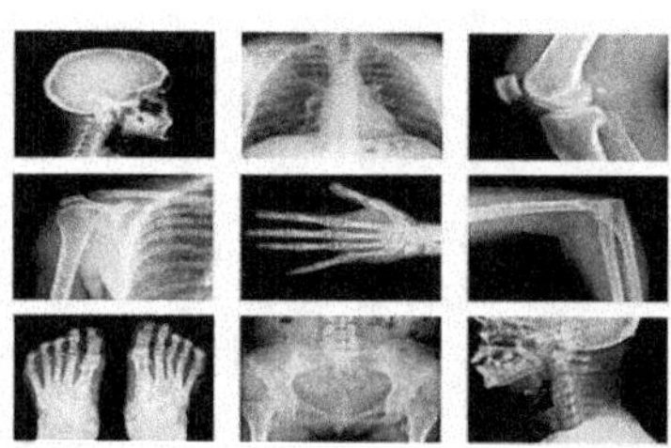

- Ultrasound.

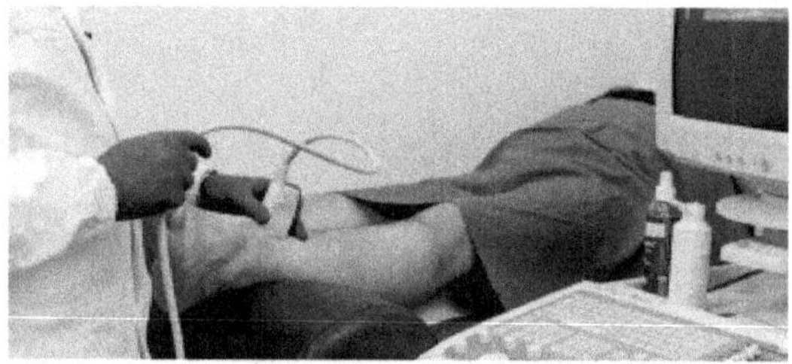

- Magnetic resonance imaging (MRI).

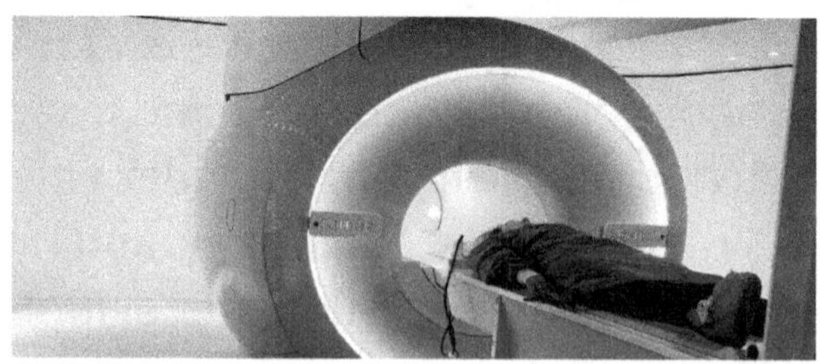

- A CT (computed tomography) scan — specifically a dual-energy CT scan.

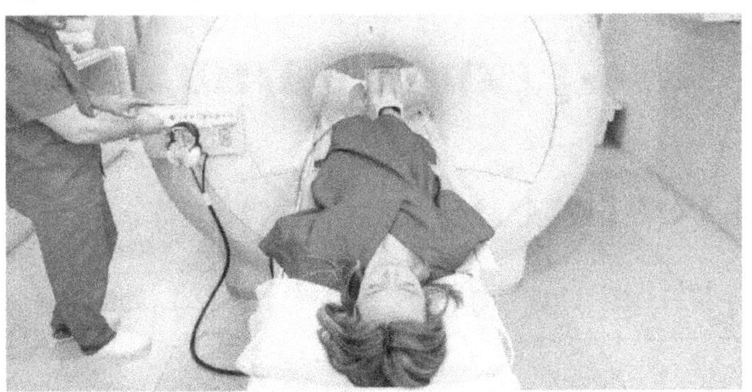

Other common tests to diagnose gout include:
- Blood tests to measure the uric acid in your blood.

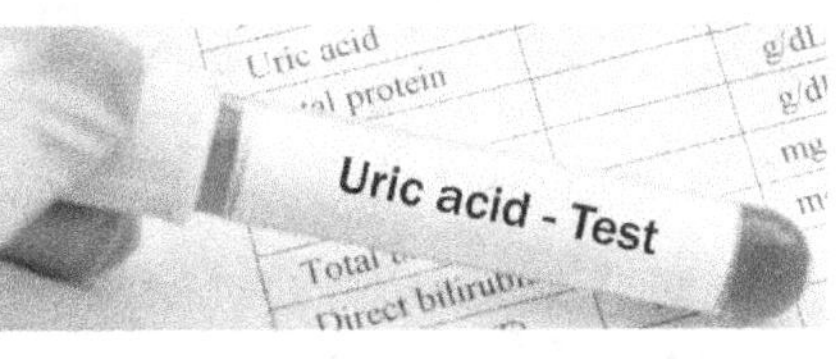

- Joint aspiration — using a needle to remove a sample of fluid from inside a joint.

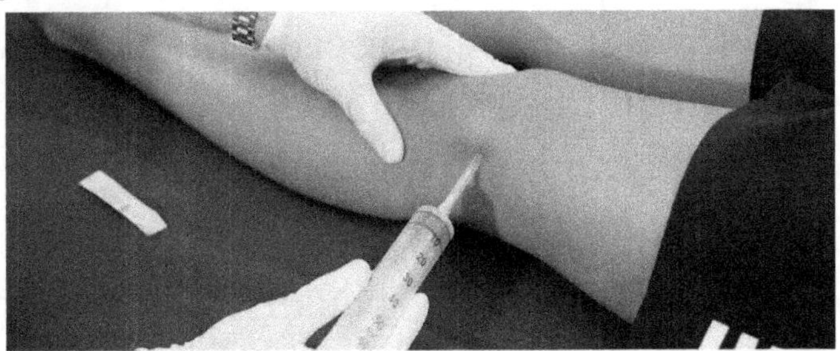

Section 5

Management and Treatment

Treatment of Gout

Getting treatment within 24 hours of a gout 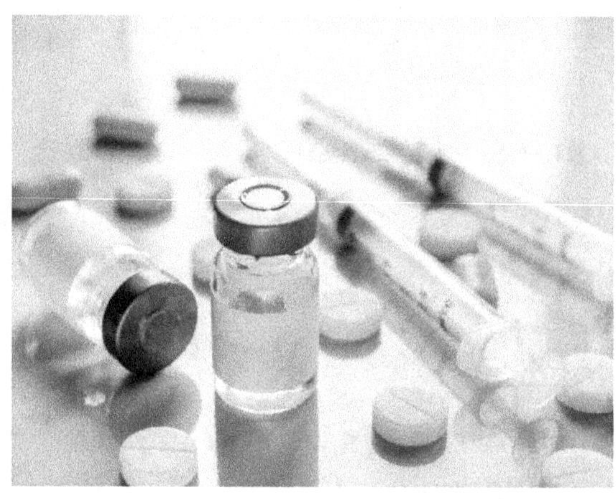 attack can help to reduce its length and severity. If you experience a sudden bout of gout attack, let your doctor know as soon as possible. Your doctor may then prescribe medication, conduct a joint fluid test or inject medication to relieve the inflammation quickly.

Treating gout is usually a combination of managing your symptoms during a flare and reducing how often you consume high-purine foods and drinks.

Managing Gout with a Healthy Diet

Adopting a gout-friendly diet that is low in purines can greatly reduce our risk of developing gout and the frequency of gout attacks. Eating lots of fruit and vegetables and avoiding the foods known to contribute to gout are great ways to maintain a healthy weight, an important way to prevent gout, and to stay healthy all-round.

Here are some foods that can help to prevent or manage gout, and foods that persons with gout should avoid.

☑ Foods that help to prevent gout include:

Carbohydrates

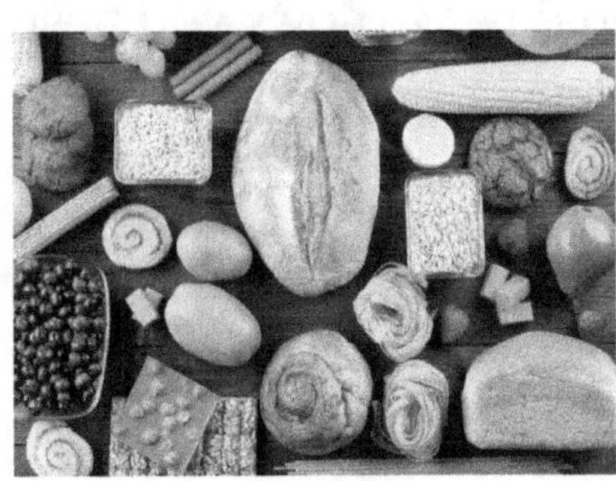

Staples such as rice, potatoes, corn-based foods, and wheat-based foods like bread can help to reduce our risk of gout. The best kind of carbohydrates to choose for all-round health and to prevent gout are complex carbohydrates. Complex carbohydrates such as wholegrain foods and brown rice take longer for the body to break down and improve gut and cardiovascular health.

Water

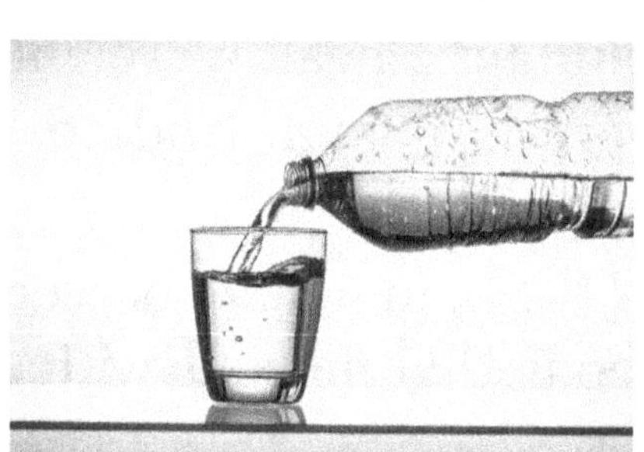

Drinking plenty of fluids is important to reduce the impact of gout, as well as to boost general health and kidney function. Most people should aim to drink 8 eight-ounce glasses of water a day – that's around 2 liters. However, if your doctor has told you to limit your fluid intake, it's important to follow the advice of the healthcare professional who knows you best.

Fruit and vegetables

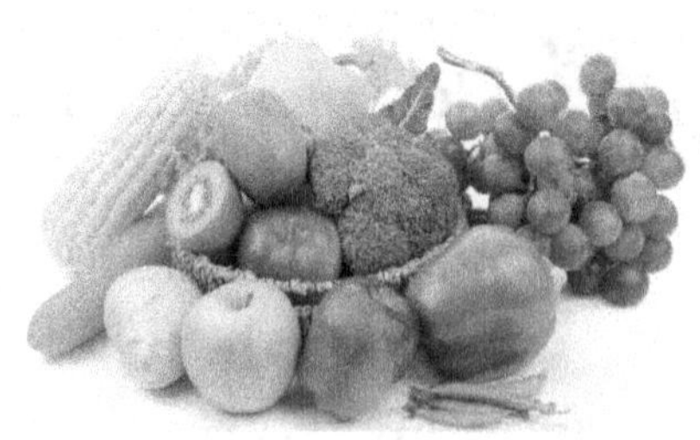

A healthy diet should contain a wide variety of fruits and vegetables to maintain overall health and lower the risk of gout.

Lean meat

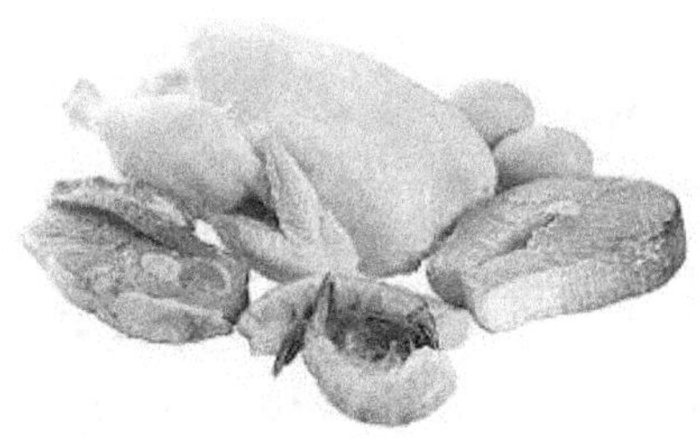

Whenever possible, choose fish, poultry, low-fat dairy, and plant-based proteins over high-fat meats such as beef.

☑ Foods to avoid include;

Red meat

Reducing your intake of meat, especially purine-rich meat, can significantly reduce your risk of developing gout.

Organ meats (offal)

Liver, kidneys, sweetbreads and other organ meats are also known to trigger gout and gout attacks.

Seafood

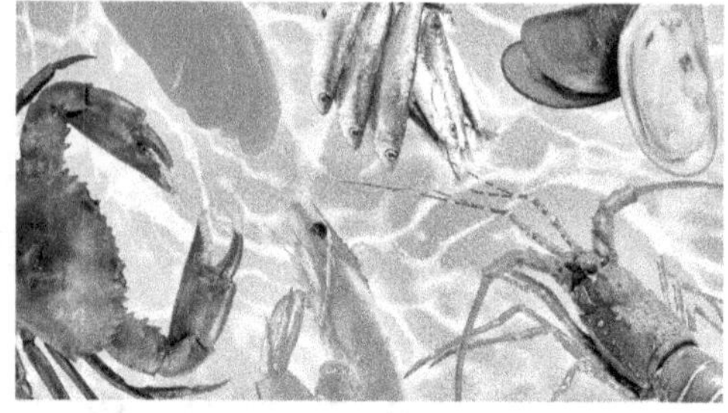

Shellfish, anchovies and sardines in particular are high in gout-causing purines. However, moderation is key as fishes do have many other health benefits.

Alcohol

Drinking alcohol is one of the most well-known triggers for gout. Certain types of alcohol seem to carry the most risk – beer and strong spirits particularly – but avoiding or reducing alcohol intake in general is recommended for people prone to gout, especially during a flare-up.

Fructose

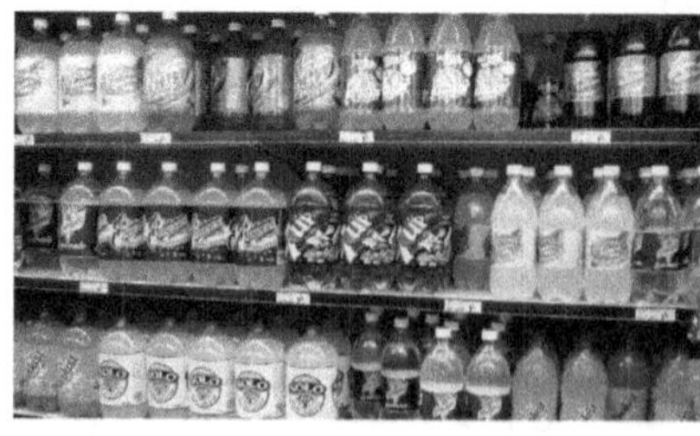

Fructose is a sugar found in fruit that's closely linked to gout risk. Foods that are highest in fructose are sugary soft drinks, juices and heavily processed sugars like corn syrup. While fruit itself does contain fructose, it is still an important part of a healthy diet. Hence, those with gout should continue to eat fruit in moderation but avoid processed sugars and soda as much as possible.

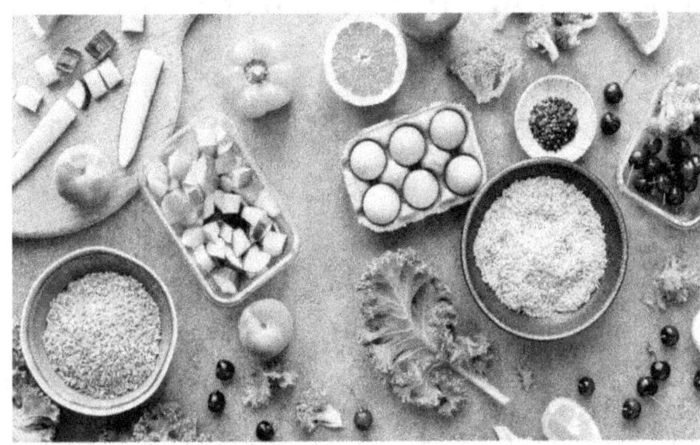 Studies have shown that people who eat eggs, dairy products and plant-based foods had the lowest risk of gout, and while people who followed a strictly plant-based diet were slightly more prone to gout, the group that ate the most meat were at significantly higher risk.

If you're looking to reduce your meat intake, vegetarian meat alternatives are available, but some are better than others at reducing gout risk. Mycoprotein-based foods such as Quorn™ and soya proteins are relatively higher in purines compared to wheat or egg-based proteins.

Potential Complications of Untreated Gout

If left untreated, gout can cause long-term damage to the joints and has the potential to be harmful and debilitating. Without proper management, a gout attack can become serious and cause permanent damage to the joint.

The ongoing inflammation and build-up of irritant crystals in the joints of a person with gout can increase their risk of joint infection. As the symptoms of joint infection can easily be confused as a mere gout attack, people often are unaware that their joint is infected, resulting in delayed treatment. This can lead to septic arthritis, a potentially life-threatening condition.

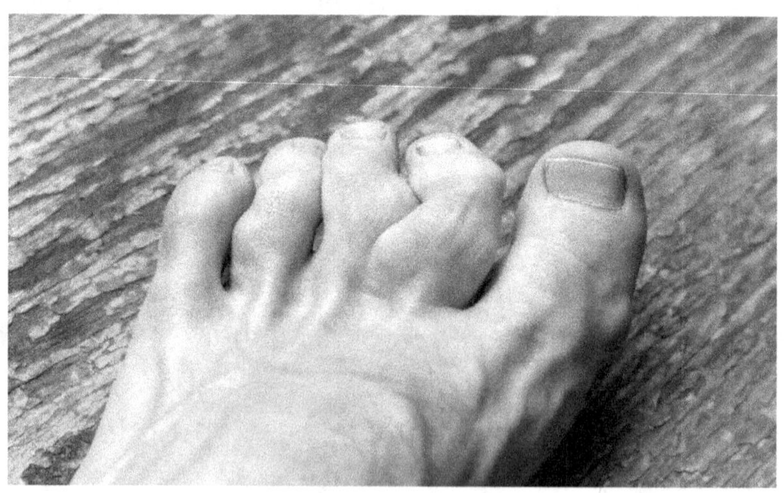

Section 6

Medications for Gout

While a healthy diet and lifestyle are great ways to prevent gout and many other diseases, people who experience attacks of gout may also be prescribed medications. Some medications are taken long-term to reduce the risk of recurrent attacks, while others are to be taken during a gout attack.

Your healthcare provider might suggest medications to help manage your symptoms, including:

Medications for long-term gout prevention

Long-term medications are usually prescribed to lower the amount of uric acid in the body. They work by either reducing the amount of uric acid produced or controlling the way it's expelled from the body. The most common medications for long-term gout treatment are taken in pill form, and include:

- ➤ **Allopurinol** reduces the amount of uric acid the body produces. It is not usually started during an acute attack of gout – it can make a flare-up worse, although in the long run it reduces the risk of further attacks.

- ➤ **Febuxostat** works in a similar way to allopurinol to prevent the body from producing as much uric acid.

- ➤ **Probenecid** helps to increase the amount of uric acid expelled by the kidneys, reducing the amount in the body.

- ➤ **Pegloticase:** Pegloticase injection is used to treat chronic gout in adult patients who have already been treated with other medicines that did not work well. Gout is a condition that is caused by too much uric acid in the blood (hyperuricemia). Pegloticase injection works by causing less uric acid to be produced by the body.

Your doctor may recommend taking medication everyday to prevent gout. This may mean taking it even when you're not experiencing symptoms of gout. After all, prevention is always better than cure.

Medications for acute attacks of gout

Painful attacks of gout are usually managed with anti-inflammatory medication – medicines that help to reduce swelling. These kinds of medicines are sometimes known as 'NSAIDs'.Ibuprofen is the most common NSAID, which may come under the brand name Nurofen.

Here are some of the common medication prescribed for gout attacks:

- **NSAIDs:** Over-the-counter (OTC) NSAIDs, like ibuprofen and naproxen, can reduce pain and swelling during a gout attack. Some people with kidney disease, stomach ulcers and other health problems shouldn't take NSAIDs. Talk to your provider before taking NSAIDs.

- **Colchicine** is another medicine commonly used in an attack of gout. Colchicine and ibuprofen can both cause some side effects, hence are usually only recommended for a short period of time, or in low doses for longer-term management. While aspirin has anti-inflammatory properties, it is not recommended for treating gout. However, if you have to take aspirin for another reason, such as to manage heart disease or stroke risk, it's important to keep taking it unless a doctor tells you not to.

➢ **Corticosteroids:** Corticosteroids are prescription medications that reduce inflammation. Your provider might prescribe oral (by mouth) pills. They may also inject corticosteroids into your affected joints or into a muscle near your joint (intramuscularly).

Low purine diet for gout

Your healthcare provider may suggest you follow a low-purine diet. A low-purine diet encourages you to consume fewer foods and drinks with high purine content. This will help reduce uric acid in your body. It also encourages you to eat some select foods that may reduce your uric acid levels.

Section 7

Gout Attack

A severe attack of gout, known as 'acute gout' or a 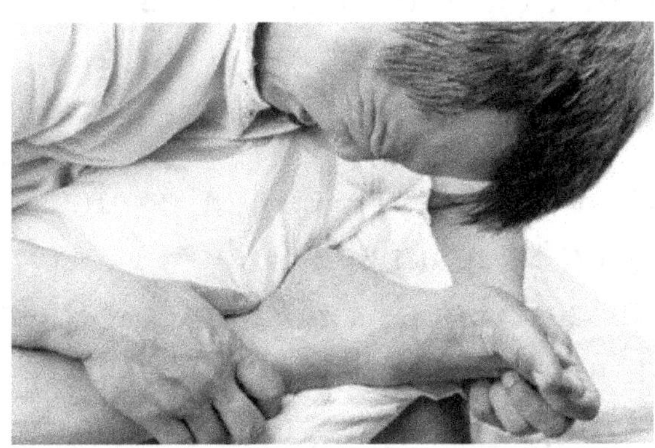 'flare up' of gout can come on suddenly. However, people can often go for long periods between attacks. Gout attacks sometimes seem to be brought on by periods of stress or other illness. People who are prone to gout might find that an attack can come on after banging the affected joints, such as after bumping an elbow or bruising a knee.

In a severe attack of gout, the pain and difficulty of using the affected joints can have a serious impact on your life, affecting mobility, sleep, and your ability to perform day-to-day tasks. Simply living with pain can have its own adverse effects on both physical and mental well-being.

Preventing Gout Attack

Those who are more likely to develop gout due to non-modifiable risk factors such as gender or family history should take extra care in managing the risk factors you can control. Adjusting your diet and maintaining a healthy weight can not only help to prevent gout, but also reduce your risk of other diseases.

Diet is the key to preventing gout. Gout sufferers should keep an eye on how much food they eat each day. Foods that increase the risk of attacks should be avoided by them. Physical activity is strongly encouraged because losing weight can also be very beneficial. But maintaining a healthy weight and diet won't prevent gout complications; medication will still be required to reach the target uric acid level.

☑ Role of Diet

Dietary control in gout patients is most helpful for those who were just starting medication to lower their level of uric acid. They should try to avoid eating large quantities of foods that are high in purines. These foods are not to be removed completely from the diet but consumed in moderation:

> Red meat, game and offal such as venison, kidneys, rabbit and liver

> Seafood, particularly oily fish such as anchovies, herrings and sardines as well as shellfish like mussels and crabs

> Foods rich in yeast extracts such as Marmite, Bovril and Vegemite

> Processed foods and drinks such as nuggets, sausages and carbonated drinks

> All types of alcohol cause more uric acid to be reabsorbed by the kidneys, raising blood uric acid levels. Beer, in particular, has a high purine level and so contributes to blood uric acid elevation. However, drinking a bit of wine does not appear to increase the risk of triggering an attack.

While the foods that contain a high level of purines will put you at a high risk of gout, there are so many other foods in different categories that can help you keep gout complications in check:

> **Water** – Drinking at least two liters of water a day will help decrease the chance

of stones forming if you have gout and a history of kidney stones,

➤ **Fruit** – While fruit and fresh fruit juices contain sugar, the benefits of eating fruit outweigh the negatives. Instead, try reducing how much sugar you consume from other sources

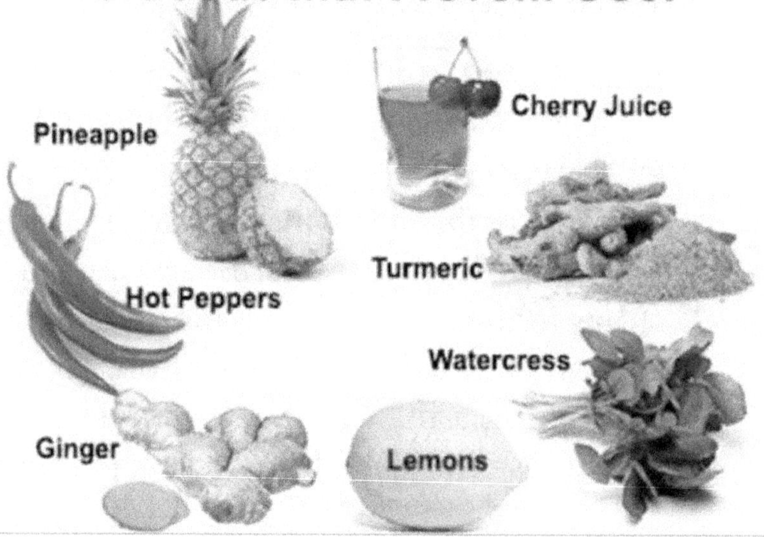

➤ **Protein-rich foods** – Protein is an important part of your diet commonly sourced from meat and fish. Just stick to your diet and get your protein from other sources like soybeans, eggs, lentils or dairy products instead.

➢ **Vitamin C** – Make sure your diet includes plenty of fruit and vegetables. Research has shown that vitamin C may slightly reduce uric acid levels in people with gout. If you are considering taking vitamin C supplements, ask your doctor if the vitamin C supplements could interact with other medications.

➢ **Cherries** – Research has shown that cherries may reduce the risk of having an acute attack of gout, particularly when taken with allopurinol.

➢ **Skimmed milk and low-fat yogurt** – Drinking skimmed milk and eating low-fat yogurt may help to prevent attacks of gout.

➢ **Oatmeal, wheat germ, and bran** – These particular sources of carbohydrates contain moderate levels of purine but are not significant gout risk factors.

☑ Physical Activity

Being overweight has been connected to gout. To control the danger of this ailment, diet and physical activity are highly suggested. Exercise is beneficial to your overall health and

wellbeing in addition to lowering your risk of
having   an   attack.

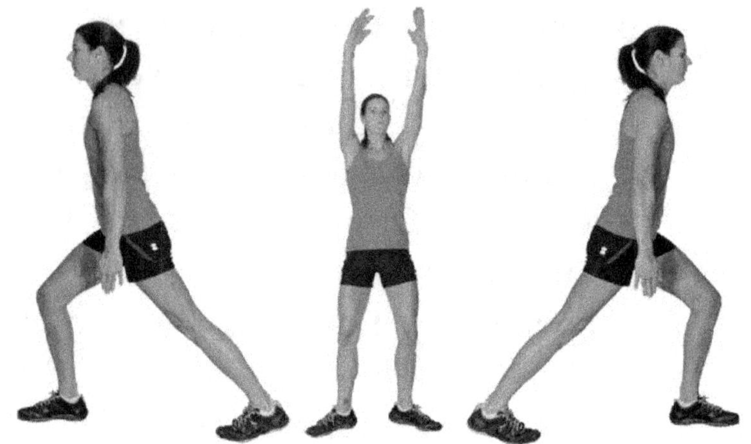

Patients with established gout should follow a
low-impact exercise program, particularly if
X-rays show foot joint damage. Increase your
workload gradually until you are completing
sessions on a regular basis.

You can work longer and harder at what you're
doing as your confidence grows. Just keep in
mind that exercising while experiencing a gout
flare-up is never a smart idea since it could
make the discomfort worse. After the
discomfort and swelling have decreased, it's
crucial to take some time off and heal before
returning to your workout routine.

Burning calories is especially beneficial from
exercises that cause dyspnea.

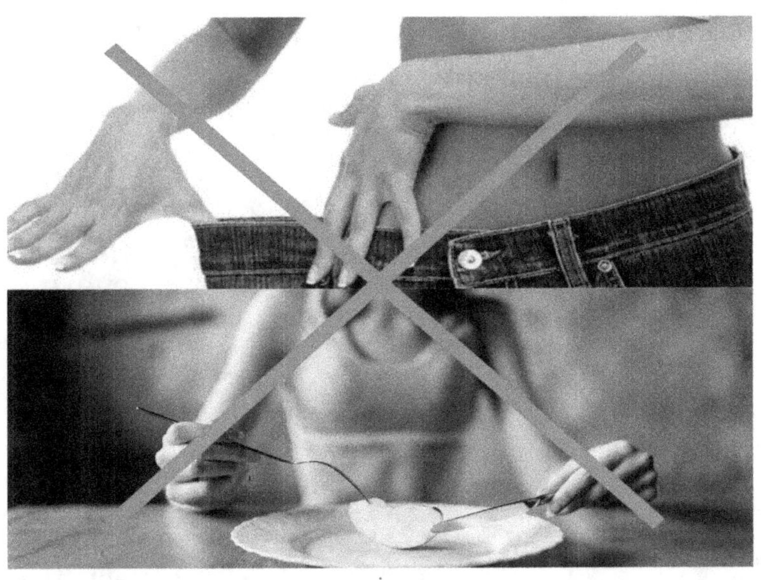

Severe weight loss or starvation diets should be avoided as they can cause your body to break down cells more quickly, which can boost urate levels. Alternatively, engage in enjoyable physical pursuits like dance, brisk walking, or doubles tennis. Finding an activity or sport that you enjoy and can stick with is helpful. While some individuals prefer to be outside and breathe in the fresh air, others find it fun and motivating to join a sports club or the gym.

For gout patients, the emotional effects of this condition can be just as impactful as the physical symptoms.

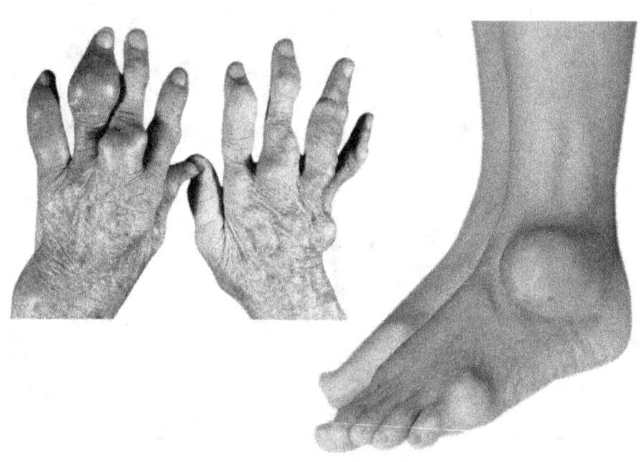

Long term damage and severe pain from the attacks of gout can affect your daily life, resulting in insomnia and affecting mental health. From time to time, your gout may get on top of you. With the help of a professional carer in the comfort of your own home, you can recover better and maintain your wellbeing for much longer.

Living with Gout

If left untreated, gout can be a very painful condition that might have long-term consequences. People who suffer from gout frequently have many health issues because the risk factors for gout are also associated with other major diseases.

Without gout, as with other health issues or mobility issues that reduces our ability to care for ourselves, it can occasionally be challenging to carry on leading the kind of life we enjoy. When we only need a little additional help at home or to get outside, having committed and qualified home caregivers can provide us with the support we need to get through challenging times. You can continue to lead the fulfilling, active, and healthy lifestyle that you deserve when you receive high-quality care in the comfort of your own home.